APPLIED GCP IN CLINICAL TRIALS

A Practical Guide for Every Step

Dr Essam Abdelhakim

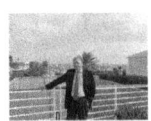

Copyright © 2024 Dr Essam Abdelhakim

All rights reserved

The characters and events portrayed in this book are fictitious. Any similarity to real persons, living or dead, is coincidental and not intended by the author.

No part of this book may be reproduced, or stored in a retrieval system, or transmitted in any form or by any means, electronic, mechanical, photocopying, recording, or otherwise, without express written permission of the publisher.

Cover design by: Art Painter
Library of Congress Control Number: 2018675309
Printed in the United States of America

CONTENTS

Title Page
Copyright
Introduction
Chapter 1: Introduction to GCP and Clinical Trials   1
Chapter 2: Trial Planning and Protocol Development   8
Chapter 3: Site Selection and Initiation   16
Chapter 4: Informed Consent Process   24
Chapter 5: Participant Recruitment and Retention   32
Chapter 6: Conducting the Trial: Day-to-Day Operations   39
Chapter 7: Adverse Events and Safety Reporting   45
Chapter 8: Monitoring Clinical Trials   51
Chapter 9: Quality Management and Audits   58
Chapter 10: Data Management and Integrity   64
Chapter 11: Investigational Medicinal Product (IMP) Management   69
Chapter 12: Closing a Clinical Trial   75
Chapter 13: Post-Trial Considerations   80
Chapter 14: Case Studies in GCP Application   85
Chapter 15: Emerging Trends in GCP and Future Directions   89
About The Author   95

INTRODUCTION

Applied GCP is more than just following a checklist of regulatory requirements, it is about safeguarding participant welfare, ensuring data quality, and maintaining the credibility of clinical research.

As clinical trials become increasingly global and complex, stakeholders must continuously evolve their practices to meet emerging challenges while upholding the highest standards of ethics and science.

Through the chapters and **case studies** in this book, you will gain a deeper understanding of how to implement GCP in practical settings, ensuring that your trials are conducted efficiently, ethically, and in compliance with the ever-changing clinical research environment.

This book will serve as a practical, hands-on resource throughout your clinical trial journey, offering solutions, strategies, and lessons learned from real-world experiences in the field of clinical research.

CHAPTER 1: INTRODUCTION TO GCP AND CLINICAL TRIALS

Overview of GCP Principles (Focus on Practical Relevance)

Good Clinical Practice (GCP) is an internationally recognized ethical and scientific quality standard for designing, conducting, recording, and reporting clinical trials involving human subjects.

It ensures that the rights, safety, and well-being of trial participants are protected, and that clinical trial data is credible and accurate.

In practice, GCP principles are embedded into the daily workings of clinical trials, affecting every aspect of the trial from planning to reporting. Adherence to GCP is not just a regulatory requirement but is vital for ensuring trust between stakeholders, ensuring the scientific integrity of the trial, and safeguarding the welfare of patients.

Here are some key GCP principles, explained with a practical focus on their application:

1. **Ethics and Participant Safety**:
   Every clinical trial must be conducted in accordance with the Declaration of Helsinki, ensuring that the rights, safety, and well-being of participants are prioritized. This principle applies to all stakeholders involved in patient interactions. For example, an investigator must obtain informed consent before any trial-related procedure is performed.

2. **Informed Consent**:
   One of the core tenets of GCP is that participants must voluntarily provide informed consent after being fully

educated about the risks, benefits, and alternatives related to the clinical trial. Practically, this means that clinical staff must be trained to clearly explain the trial and ensure participants fully understand their involvement.

3. **Data Integrity and Confidentiality**:
GCP mandates that data generated during the trial must be accurate, reliable, and handled with confidentiality. From source documentation to final data entries in Case Report Forms (CRFs), there should be a clear chain of custody for all information, ensuring that data is credible and properly recorded.

4. **Protocol Adherence**:
The protocol acts as the blueprint of the clinical trial, detailing all trial procedures and methods. GCP stresses strict adherence to this protocol. In practical terms, this means all stakeholders—investigators, study coordinators, monitors—must be familiar with the protocol and understand that any deviation requires documentation and justification.

5. **Quality Assurance and Control**:
GCP requires quality systems to be in place throughout the trial process. Practically, this translates into routine monitoring, audits, and inspections to ensure compliance with the trial protocol, SOPs (Standard Operating Procedures), and regulatory requirements.

By focusing on these principles, clinical trial teams can ensure compliance with GCP, helping to safeguard participants and maintain the credibility of the trial's findings.

Roles And Responsibilities Of Stakeholders

A clinical trial involves multiple stakeholders, each with a distinct role and set of responsibilities under GCP. Understanding these roles helps maintain the smooth operation of the trial and ensures compliance with regulations.

1. **Investigators**:
    The investigator, typically a physician or clinician, is responsible for the overall conduct of the trial at the site. Key responsibilities include:
    - Ensuring the trial is conducted according to the approved protocol.
    - Obtaining informed consent from participants.
    - Reporting adverse events promptly.
    - Maintaining accurate trial documentation and ensuring data quality.

    In practice, investigators must work closely with the study team and monitors to ensure compliance with the trial protocol and GCP guidelines. For example, they must document any protocol deviations and explain how they will be corrected to prevent future occurrences.

2. **Sponsor**:
    The sponsor is the organization or individual responsible for initiating, managing, and financing the clinical trial. The sponsor's responsibilities include:
    - Designing and approving the clinical trial protocol.
    - Selecting qualified investigators and trial sites.
    - Providing necessary resources, including trial materials and training.
    - Ensuring data monitoring and quality control throughout the trial.

    Sponsors must ensure that trials are conducted ethically

and in compliance with regulatory requirements. They often delegate operational aspects of trial management to Contract Research Organizations (CROs) while retaining ultimate responsibility.

3. **Contract Research Organization (CRO)**:

    A CRO is a company contracted by the sponsor to perform some or all trial-related duties and functions. CROs play a crucial role in managing the day-to-day operations of a clinical trial, including:

    - Site monitoring and management.
    - Regulatory submissions.
    - Data management and statistical analysis.

CROs must follow the same GCP principles as sponsors, particularly when it comes to trial monitoring and data integrity.

4. **Institutional Review Board (IRB)/Ethics Committee (EC)**:

    The IRB or EC is an independent body responsible for reviewing and approving the trial protocol to ensure the ethical conduct of the trial. Their key responsibilities include:

    - Protecting the rights and welfare of trial participants.
    - Reviewing informed consent forms and participant-facing materials.
    - Monitoring trial conduct, particularly in cases of adverse events or protocol deviations.

In practical terms, the IRB/EC serves as an oversight body to ensure that the trial does not expose participants to unnecessary risk and that it is ethically justified.

5. **Monitors**:

    Monitors, often working on behalf of the sponsor or

CRO, are responsible for ensuring that the trial is conducted according to the protocol and GCP. Their duties include:

- Reviewing data for accuracy and completeness.
- Identifying and reporting protocol deviations.
- Conducting site visits to ensure compliance with trial procedures.

Practically, monitors serve as a bridge between the sponsor and the trial site, ensuring that all stakeholders are following the appropriate guidelines and maintaining data integrity.

Regulatory Framework And Guidelines

The regulatory framework for clinical trials is governed by various international and national guidelines. The key global GCP guideline is the **International Council for Harmonisation (ICH) E6 Good Clinical Practice (GCP)** guideline, which harmonizes regulations across different regions.

This guideline applies to all trials that aim for regulatory approval in major regions like the USA, EU, and Japan.

In addition to ICH GCP, the following regulatory authorities provide region-specific guidance:

- **FDA (U.S. Food and Drug Administration)**: Oversees clinical trials conducted in the United States. The FDA has its own set of regulations, outlined in Title 21 of the Code of Federal Regulations (CFR), particularly 21 CFR Parts 50, 54, 56, 312, and 812, covering informed consent, IRBs, and investigational drug/device trials.
- **EMA (European Medicines Agency)**: Governs clinical trials within the European Union and follows the EU Clinical Trials Regulation.

- **MHRA (Medicines and Healthcare products Regulatory Agency)**: Responsible for overseeing clinical trials in the UK.

For stakeholders, understanding the applicable regulatory requirements is essential for ensuring that trials are not only scientifically sound but also legally compliant.

Case Study: Identifying Stakeholder Roles In A Complex Global Clinical Trial

Background:
A pharmaceutical company is conducting a global phase III clinical trial for a new oncology drug. The trial involves multiple countries, including the U.S., EU, and Asia, and requires collaboration between a sponsor, CRO, IRBs, and multiple investigative sites.

Challenge:
The trial faced delays due to protocol deviations, missed safety reporting deadlines, and inadequate data collection in several sites.

The sponsor received a warning from the U.S. FDA and was under pressure to correct these issues while the trial was ongoing.

Stakeholder Roles And Actions:

- **Sponsor**: The sponsor assumed ultimate responsibility for the trial and immediately engaged the CRO to address the identified issues. They also increased monitoring frequency at underperforming sites and provided additional resources for site training.
- **CRO**: The CRO was responsible for overseeing daily operations, including monitoring and data collection. Upon realizing the magnitude of protocol deviations,

the CRO increased site monitoring visits, retrained site staff, and reviewed data management procedures to improve accuracy.

- **Investigators**: Investigators at various sites were required to immediately report any deviations or adverse events. Some sites failed to do so, leading to a need for retraining on GCP principles, particularly on the importance of timely safety reporting.
- **IRB/EC**: IRBs were alerted to the deviations and required a thorough review of the protocol to determine if amendments were necessary. They also requested more frequent safety monitoring updates.
- **Monitors**: Monitors were crucial in identifying issues with data integrity and promptly reported these issues to the sponsor and CRO. They implemented corrective and preventive actions, ensuring that subsequent site visits focused on resolving the problem areas.

Outcome:

Through enhanced communication between stakeholders and implementation of corrective measures, the trial resumed normal operations.

Key GCP principles such as protocol adherence and timely reporting were reinforced, and a revised monitoring plan ensured future compliance.

This case study highlights the critical importance of each stakeholder understanding their roles and the practical application of GCP in resolving complex issues during a trial.

CHAPTER 2: TRIAL PLANNING AND PROTOCOL DEVELOPMENT

Effective trial planning is one of the most critical phases in a clinical trial. A well-thought-out protocol sets the foundation for the entire study, ensuring that the trial is conducted ethically, efficiently, and in compliance with regulatory guidelines.

Understanding Protocol Design And Feasibility (Focus On Ensuring Protocol Adherence)

The protocol is the central document of any clinical trial, outlining the study's objectives, design, methodology, statistical considerations, and operational details. Developing a protocol that is scientifically sound, ethically appropriate, and operationally feasible is crucial for the success of a clinical trial.

Key Elements Of A Clinical Trial Protocol

1. **Study Objectives**:
   Clearly define the primary and secondary objectives of the trial. For instance, in a phase III oncology trial, the primary objective might be to assess the overall survival rate, while secondary objectives may include evaluating progression-free survival or quality of life. Clear objectives help maintain focus throughout the trial.

2. **Study Design**:
   The design includes the type of study (e.g., randomized controlled trial, double-blind, placebo-controlled), the population being studied, and the duration of the trial. It also includes details on interventions, dosing regimens, and endpoints. The design should ensure that the study is scientifically valid and that results can be reproduced.

3. **Inclusion and Exclusion Criteria**:
   These criteria are essential for selecting participants and ensuring that the study population is appropriate for the research question. Practical application of these criteria involves ensuring that investigative sites can recruit patients that match the outlined criteria without difficulty.

4. **Study Procedures and Assessments**:
   Detailed descriptions of all study procedures (e.g., lab tests, physical exams, imaging) should be included, with timelines for assessments. A practical focus would be ensuring that investigative sites have the capacity to perform these assessments as required by the protocol.

5. **Statistical Considerations**:
   A statistical plan should outline the methods for data analysis, sample size calculations, and statistical tests to be used. A feasibility check ensures that the study can recruit enough participants to meet statistical power requirements within the given timeframe.

Ensuring Protocol Adherence

While designing a protocol, one of the key challenges is ensuring that it will be adhered to throughout the trial. Protocol adherence is vital for maintaining the integrity of the data, ensuring patient safety, and reducing the likelihood of deviations.

To facilitate protocol adherence:

- **Train Investigators and Site Staff**: Make sure that all staff involved in the trial fully understand the protocol. This can be achieved through regular training sessions and workshops. Complex protocols often require ongoing support and clarification.
- **Simplify Procedures Where Possible**: While scientific rigor is necessary, simplifying procedures (e.g., reducing unnecessary tests or visits) can increase adherence, especially at busy trial sites.
- **Monitor Adherence**: Monitors should regularly check that the protocol is being followed. Early detection of deviations allows for timely corrective actions.

Regulatory Submissions And Approvals (Navigating The Approval Process)

Once the protocol is developed, it needs to undergo a regulatory approval process before the clinical trial can commence. Regulatory bodies ensure that the trial complies with ethical guidelines and that participant safety is prioritized.

Each country has its own regulatory authority (e.g., FDA in the U.S., EMA in Europe), but most operate under the framework of ICH GCP guidelines.

Key Steps In Regulatory Submissions:

1. **Preparation of Regulatory Dossier**:
   The regulatory dossier includes the trial protocol, investigator's brochure, informed consent forms, and other essential documents like the investigational product dossier. Preparing these documents requires close coordination between the sponsor and investigators to ensure that all the information

provided is accurate and complete.
2. **Navigating the Approval Process**:
    - **Institutional Review Board (IRB) or Ethics Committee (EC)**: Before any regulatory submission, the protocol must first be approved by an IRB or EC. These bodies review the ethical aspects of the trial and ensure that participant rights and safety are protected.
    - **Competent Authorities (e.g., FDA, EMA)**: In parallel with IRB/EC approval, the trial must also be submitted to the relevant regulatory authority for review. The submission includes not only the protocol but also documents related to the investigational product, investigator qualifications, and trial management plans.
3. **Managing Queries and Amendments**:
Regulatory authorities may ask questions or request amendments to the protocol. Sponsors and investigators need to be prepared to address these queries promptly. Often, clarifications are needed around risk/benefit assessments, patient safety measures, or statistical justifications. Addressing these effectively can accelerate the approval process.
4. **Approval Timeline**:
Approval timelines vary depending on the region and the complexity of the trial. Regulatory authorities often follow strict timelines for processing applications, but sponsors must be prepared for possible delays and plan accordingly.

Key Considerations For A Successful Submission:

- **Thorough Documentation**: Ensure that all necessary documents, including the Investigator's Brochure, informed consent forms, and trial-specific forms, are properly completed and submitted.
- **Local Requirements**: Each country may have additional specific requirements, such as additional forms or safety data. Ensure compliance with local regulations.
- **Ongoing Communication**: Regular communication with regulatory bodies can facilitate a smoother approval process. Sponsors should establish a point of contact to address regulatory questions or requests for more information promptly.

Budgeting And Resource Planning

A well-developed clinical trial budget ensures that all aspects of the trial are adequately funded, from protocol development through to trial closeout. Proper resource planning also helps prevent delays and enables efficient trial execution.

Steps For Budgeting And Resource Allocation:

1. **Cost of Protocol Development**:
   The costs associated with protocol development include expenses for protocol design, consultations with experts, and pre-trial feasibility assessments. Sponsors must ensure that resources are available for this phase, particularly if the protocol requires amendments or revisions.
2. **Site Budgeting**:
   Every trial site incurs costs for enrolling participants, conducting study-related procedures, and monitoring participants. Site budgets typically cover:

- Investigator fees
- Staff salaries
- Administrative expenses (e.g., IRB submissions, recruitment advertising)
- Costs of trial-related tests and procedures

Negotiating fair compensation for sites helps to ensure they have the necessary resources to conduct the trial effectively.

3. **Investigational Product and Logistics**:
   Resource planning includes budgeting for the manufacture, storage, and distribution of investigational products. This must also account for any specific storage requirements, such as temperature-controlled environments, as well as potential delays in shipping.

4. **Monitoring and Auditing**:
   GCP requires regular monitoring of trial sites, which incurs costs related to travel, accommodation, and personnel time. Sponsors should also account for periodic audits, which ensure trial conduct is in compliance with the protocol and regulatory requirements.

5. **Contingency Planning**:
   Unexpected events, such as recruitment challenges or adverse event reporting, can increase trial costs. Sponsors should allocate contingency funds to accommodate these unforeseen expenses without compromising the trial's progress.

Effective Resource Allocation:

- **Outsourcing to CROs**: Outsourcing trial management to a Contract Research Organization (CRO) can be cost-effective, but the sponsor must ensure that the CRO has

adequate resources and expertise to manage the trial successfully.
- **Technology Investments**: Investing in trial management software, eCRFs (electronic case report forms), and other digital tools can streamline data collection and reduce the time and cost of monitoring.

Case Study: Developing A Feasible Clinical Trial Protocol And Gaining Ethics Approval

Background:
A sponsor is developing a global phase II trial investigating a new diabetes medication. The trial involves multiple countries and targets diverse populations, including patients with co-existing conditions like cardiovascular disease.

During the trial planning phase, the sponsor faced challenges in designing a feasible protocol that could be approved by ethics committees in multiple regions.

Challenges:
1. **Protocol Complexity**: The original protocol required 12 in-person visits over 6 months, multiple invasive tests, and strict inclusion criteria that limited the pool of eligible participants.
2. **Budget Constraints**: The initial budget underestimated the costs of participant recruitment, particularly in regions with lower healthcare access.
3. **Ethical Concerns**: IRBs in some countries raised concerns about the invasive tests, questioning their necessity for participant safety and the overall research objectives.

Actions Taken:
- **Protocol Revision**: The sponsor worked with key opinion leaders to revise the protocol, reducing the

number of in-person visits to 8 by using telemedicine for routine check-ins and simplifying the testing schedule to non-invasive assessments wherever possible.

- **Feasibility Study**: Before finalizing the protocol, the sponsor conducted a feasibility study with selected trial sites to ensure that they could enroll enough patients to meet statistical power requirements. This study revealed that sites in rural areas would need extra resources to manage recruitment and follow-up.
- **Resource Adjustment**: To address budget constraints, the sponsor reallocated resources to increase the participant compensation and support transportation costs in rural areas, ensuring that recruitment goals could be met.
- **Ethics Approval**: After revising the protocol to reduce the number of invasive tests, the IRBs provided approval, with the condition that regular safety monitoring be implemented to ensure participant safety during remote assessments.

Outcome:
By focusing on feasibility and addressing IRB concerns early, the sponsor was able to secure ethics approval and proceed with the trial. The revised protocol not only improved participant compliance but also reduced overall trial costs by minimizing unnecessary procedures.

This case demonstrates the importance of flexibility in protocol development and the need to address both scientific and practical concerns during the trial planning phase.

CHAPTER 3: SITE SELECTION AND INITIATION

The success of a clinical trial depends significantly on the selection of appropriate trial sites and ensuring that each site is prepared to conduct the study according to Good Clinical Practice (GCP) standards.

Key Factors In Site Selection

Selecting the right clinical trial sites is crucial for ensuring high-quality data, efficient patient recruitment, and adherence to the protocol. The site selection process involves assessing various factors to ensure that the site has the capacity and expertise to conduct the trial successfully.

1. Capacity To Conduct The Trial

- **Patient Population**: The site must have access to a patient population that matches the study's inclusion and exclusion criteria. For example, in a trial for a rare genetic disorder, the site needs to demonstrate that it has or can recruit a sufficient number of eligible patients.
- **Facilities and Equipment**: The site should have the necessary infrastructure, such as specialized diagnostic equipment, lab facilities, and storage for investigational products. This is particularly important for trials that require complex procedures, like imaging studies or storage of biologics that require

cold chain management.
- **Staffing and Resources**: The site should have enough qualified staff, including investigators, research coordinators, and data managers, to handle the workload. Sites with previous experience in similar trials are more likely to have well-established processes and dedicated research staff.

2. Expertise And Experience

- **Principal Investigator (PI) Experience**: The experience and qualifications of the PI are paramount. Ideally, the PI should have previous experience in conducting clinical trials in the relevant therapeutic area. This ensures that they are familiar with the complexities of trial protocols, patient recruitment, and regulatory requirements.
- **Research Team Competency**: Beyond the PI, the entire research team must have the appropriate skills. This includes coordinators who handle day-to-day trial activities and data collection staff who ensure accurate documentation.
- **Past Performance**: Evaluating the site's performance in past trials can provide insight into its reliability. Metrics such as patient enrollment rates, protocol compliance, and the quality of data submitted can help determine whether the site is a good fit for the study. Sites with a history of protocol deviations or issues with data integrity may pose risks to trial timelines and outcomes.

3. Recruitment Feasibility

- **Patient Recruitment Potential**: Analyzing the site's historical recruitment performance is key. Sites that

consistently meet or exceed recruitment targets are more likely to succeed in future studies. It's also important to evaluate whether the site has implemented strategies to address recruitment challenges, such as access to referral networks or digital recruitment platforms.
- **Patient Retention**: Beyond recruitment, retention is critical. Sites with good patient engagement strategies (e.g., regular follow-up, providing detailed patient information) tend to have higher retention rates, which is crucial for long-term studies where patient drop-out can affect the integrity of the data.

4. Geographic And Cultural Considerations

- **Location**: The geographic location of the site can impact patient accessibility, regulatory requirements, and logistical aspects like the transport of investigational products. Additionally, if a trial is multinational, local regulatory requirements and healthcare standards must be considered.
- **Cultural Sensitivity**: Sites that serve diverse populations need to be culturally sensitive in patient recruitment and retention strategies. For instance, informed consent materials should be available in languages spoken by the patient population, and site staff should be trained to navigate cultural differences that may affect trial participation.

Site Initiation Visit (Siv): Ensuring Compliance From Day 1

Once a site has been selected, the Site Initiation Visit (SIV) is the next critical step to ensure that the site is ready to begin trial activities. The SIV is typically conducted by a Clinical

Research Associate (CRA) and serves to confirm that all necessary preparations have been made to conduct the trial in compliance with the protocol and GCP.

Objectives Of The Siv

1. **Review of Protocol and Study Procedures**:
   During the SIV, the CRA reviews the study protocol with the PI and the research team, emphasizing key study procedures, endpoints, and timelines. This ensures that everyone understands the trial's objectives and the specific tasks they are responsible for.

2. **Regulatory and Ethical Approvals**:
   The CRA verifies that all necessary regulatory documents, including IRB/EC approvals, have been obtained and are up to date. They will also check that the informed consent forms (ICFs) are compliant with both regulatory and ethical requirements, ensuring patient protection.

3. **Investigational Product (IP) Management**:
   Proper handling of the investigational product is critical to trial success. The CRA ensures that the site has received the IP, understands its storage requirements (e.g., temperature control), and has systems in place to track its dispensing to patients. Any issues with IP logistics can delay the trial or compromise patient safety.

4. **Data Collection and Documentation**:
   The CRA reviews the data collection process with the site staff, including how to complete case report forms (CRFs) and report adverse events. The importance of accurate, timely, and complete data is emphasized, as

this impacts both the trial's integrity and regulatory compliance.

5. **GCP and Protocol Training**:
   All site staff involved in the trial must be trained on GCP principles and the specifics of the study protocol. This includes training on how to avoid common pitfalls, such as protocol deviations, improper informed consent processes, and inadequate reporting of adverse events. Training should be documented as part of the site's regulatory binder.

SIV Checklist for Site Readiness

- **Signed Protocol and Regulatory Documents**
- **Adequate Investigational Product (IP) Supply**
- **Fully Trained Staff (documented)**
- **Set Up of Trial-Related Equipment**
- **Documented Process for Patient Recruitment and Retention**
- **Plan for Data Management and Reporting**

Training The Investigative Team

Training the investigative team is a key component of the SIV and is essential for ensuring that the site operates smoothly and in compliance with GCP guidelines.

All team members, from the PI to support staff, must understand their specific roles and how their activities contribute to the overall success of the trial.

Key Areas Of Training

1. **Study Protocol**:
   The protocol outlines the procedures to be followed, so the research team must be trained to adhere

strictly to these guidelines. Each team member should understand the rationale behind the study endpoints, assessments, and timelines.

2. **GCP Compliance**:
Training on GCP ensures that the site operates with patient safety as the top priority. This includes maintaining accurate documentation, obtaining proper informed consent, and reporting adverse events or deviations promptly.

3. **Data Management**:
The team must be proficient in the use of data collection systems, whether paper-based or electronic (eCRFs). Training should also cover procedures for monitoring data quality and correcting errors without compromising data integrity.

4. **IP Management**:
Staff must be trained in handling, storing, and dispensing the investigational product in accordance with the protocol and regulatory requirements. This includes managing accountability logs and preventing issues such as IP mismanagement or improper blinding.

5. **Patient Interaction**:
Effective patient communication is essential for recruitment, retention, and informed consent. Training should emphasize the importance of clear communication, addressing patient concerns, and maintaining confidentiality.

Case Study: Evaluating The Readiness Of A Clinical Trial Site

Background:

A mid-sized clinical trial for a new cardiovascular drug was initiated across several global sites. One site, located in a rural area, was selected due to its strong recruitment potential in underserved patient populations. However, during the SIV, concerns about the site's readiness to conduct the trial emerged.

Challenges:

1. **Limited Research Experience**:
   While the site's PI was a well-respected cardiologist, the site had minimal experience in conducting GCP-compliant clinical trials. The staff lacked experience with electronic case report forms (eCRFs), and the site had no established procedures for investigational product storage.

2. **Incomplete Regulatory Documentation**:
   At the time of the SIV, the site had yet to receive full ethics approval for the trial. The IRB had requested modifications to the informed consent forms, but the site staff had not yet submitted the revisions.

3. **Staff Shortages**:
   The site did not have a dedicated research coordinator, and the PI was splitting time between the trial and their clinical practice, raising concerns about whether the site could handle the trial workload.

Actions Taken:

1. **Enhanced Training**:
   The sponsor arranged for additional on-site training sessions, focusing on GCP, data management, and investigational product handling. The PI and site staff were walked through the electronic case report forms and other trial-specific systems.

2. **Regulatory Support**:
   The sponsor's regulatory team worked closely with the

site to expedite the submission of the revised informed consent forms to the IRB. In addition, the site was provided with templates and examples of properly completed regulatory documents.

3. **Resource Allocation**:
To address the staffing shortage, the sponsor agreed to fund a part-time research coordinator position at the site. This individual was responsible for managing day-to-day trial operations and ensuring that the trial adhered to protocol requirements.

Outcome:
With additional training and regulatory support, the site was able to begin patient recruitment within six weeks of the SIV. The new research coordinator played a key role in managing the trial, allowing the PI to focus on oversight and patient care. The trial proceeded without major deviations, and the site became one of the top recruiters in the study.

CHAPTER 4: INFORMED CONSENT PROCESS

The informed consent process is one of the most crucial aspects of conducting a clinical trial, ensuring that participants understand the study, its risks, and their rights before deciding to participate. Implementing a robust informed consent process that aligns with Good Clinical Practice (GCP) is not only a regulatory requirement but also an ethical obligation. This chapter will focus on the practical challenges faced in the informed consent process, solutions for addressing these challenges, and the importance of cultural and ethical considerations.

Implementing a Robust Informed Consent Process

The informed consent process is much more than just obtaining a signature on a document. It is an ongoing dialogue between the investigator and the participant, ensuring that the participant fully understands the trial and continues to feel comfortable with their involvement throughout the study. Here are the key components of implementing a robust process:

1. Ensuring Participant Understanding

- **Plain Language**: The informed consent form (ICF) should be written in clear, non-technical language that is easily understood by a layperson. Avoiding medical jargon ensures that participants can grasp the essential elements of the study, such as the study's purpose, procedures, risks, and benefits.

- **Interactive Discussion**: The informed consent process should involve a face-to-face discussion (or virtual meeting when appropriate) where the investigator or research staff goes over the consent form with the participant. During this conversation, participants should be encouraged to ask questions and clarify any doubts they may have.
- **Use of Visual Aids**: In some cases, visual aids such as charts, diagrams, or videos can be helpful in explaining complex procedures or risks. These tools can enhance understanding and engagement, particularly for studies involving technical or complicated interventions.

2. Addressing Participant Concerns

- **Time for Consideration**: Participants should be given ample time to consider their decision and discuss it with family members, friends, or a healthcare provider if needed. This step is critical to avoid any feelings of pressure or coercion.
- **Clear Explanation of Withdrawal Rights**: Participants must be made aware that they can withdraw from the study at any time, without any negative consequences. Emphasizing this right reassures participants that their autonomy is respected throughout the trial.
- **Full Disclosure of Risks**: While it is tempting to focus on the potential benefits of a trial, a robust informed consent process requires a clear and honest disclosure of risks. This includes not only risks related to the study treatment but also potential inconveniences (e.g., multiple visits, invasive procedures) and side effects.

3. Documenting The Process

- **Documentation of the Consent Discussion**: It is essential to document not just the signed consent form but also the discussion that took place between the participant and the investigator. Notes should include key topics discussed, any questions raised by the participant, and how these questions were addressed.
- **Re-consent for Protocol Amendments**: If there are significant changes to the protocol during the course of the trial, participants must be informed, and re-consent must be obtained. This ensures that participants are fully informed of any new risks or changes in the study's conduct.

4. Continuous Process Of Informed Consent

- **Ongoing Communication**: The informed consent process should not be a one-time event. Investigators must regularly check in with participants to ensure they are still comfortable with their participation. This is especially important in long-term studies or trials where new information about risks or benefits emerges.

Practical Challenges and Solutions in the Informed Consent Process

Even with a well-designed consent form and process, practical challenges may arise. Addressing these challenges is key to maintaining the integrity of the informed consent process and ensuring participant understanding and comfort.

1. Literacy Barriers

- **Challenge**: Some participants may have low literacy levels, making it difficult for them to read and understand the informed consent document.
- **Solution**: To address this, the research team should verbally explain the consent form in simple terms and check for understanding by asking participants to repeat the information in their own words. Use of audio or video formats for the informed consent information may also help in such situations.

2. Language Barriers

- **Challenge**: In multinational or multicultural trials, participants may not speak or read the language in which the informed consent form is written.
- **Solution**: In such cases, the consent form must be translated into the participant's native language, and a certified interpreter should be present during the consent discussion to ensure accurate communication. It is also critical that any verbal explanations are culturally sensitive and respectful of local customs.

3. Vulnerable Populations

- **Challenge**: Vulnerable populations, such as children, elderly individuals, or patients with cognitive impairments, may require additional safeguards during the informed consent process.
- **Solution**: For participants who are unable to provide consent themselves, legal guardians or family members may provide consent on their behalf. However, the study team should still attempt to explain the study to the participant in simple terms. For children, this might involve age-appropriate

language, and in some cases, obtaining "assent" from older children or adolescents.

4. Complex Study Protocols

- **Challenge**: Studies with complicated procedures or potential risks can be difficult for participants to fully comprehend.
- **Solution**: In these cases, the research team should use additional resources like videos, infographics, or staged discussions over multiple visits to gradually explain the study details. Breaking the consent process into manageable chunks allows the participant to digest information more easily and reduces the risk of overwhelming them.

Cultural And Ethical Considerations In Informed Consent

Informed consent is not just about legal and regulatory compliance; it also involves addressing cultural and ethical nuances that can impact how participants understand and engage with clinical trials.

1. Respect For Cultural Beliefs And Practices

- **Language and Communication Style**: In some cultures, indirect communication is preferred, and participants may be reluctant to ask questions or express doubts. The investigator must be sensitive to these communication styles and find ways to encourage open dialogue. Additionally, informed consent documents should be translated with cultural context in mind, using language that resonates with local norms.

- **Informed Consent in a Hierarchical Society**: In cultures with a strong hierarchical or family-based decision-making structure, individuals may defer to family elders or community leaders when making healthcare decisions. In such cases, involving family members in the informed consent process may be necessary to ensure participants feel supported in their decision-making.

2. Ethical Dilemmas In Low-Resource Settings

- **Coercion Risk**: In low-resource settings, offering incentives (monetary or otherwise) for participation can blur the lines between voluntary consent and coercion. It's crucial that incentives are proportional and not so large that they unduly influence participants to join a study against their better judgment.
- **Access to Healthcare**: Participants in trials conducted in low-resource areas may have limited access to healthcare outside the trial. In these settings, participants may feel obligated to participate in a trial in order to receive medical care, which raises ethical concerns. Investigators must ensure that participants are aware that their decision to participate will not affect their access to healthcare.

Case Study: Addressing Language Barriers And Cultural Sensitivity In Informed Consent

Background:
A large-scale clinical trial testing a new tuberculosis (TB) vaccine was initiated in several countries, including rural regions of Southeast Asia. One of the selected sites was in a small village where the primary language was a local dialect, and most

participants had little to no formal education.

The trial aimed to enroll hundreds of participants, including individuals from vulnerable populations like the elderly and children.

Challenges:

1. **Language Barriers**: The informed consent forms were initially provided in English and the national language, neither of which were commonly spoken by the village population.
2. **Low Literacy Levels**: Many potential participants had difficulty reading the consent form, even in their native dialect.
3. **Cultural Sensitivity**: In the local culture, healthcare decisions were often made collectively by the family, and participants felt uncomfortable making individual decisions without consulting family elders.

Actions Taken:

1. **Translation and Interpretation**: The sponsor provided translated informed consent forms in the local dialect and hired local interpreters who were fluent in both the dialect and the study's medical terminology. During the informed consent process, the interpreters facilitated discussions between the investigators and participants, ensuring accurate communication.
2. **Use of Audio Consent Forms**: For participants who could not read, an audio version of the informed consent form was developed. This allowed participants to listen to the form in their native dialect, with the option to replay sections for better understanding.
3. **Family Involvement**: Understanding the local decision-making structure, the research team encouraged participants to discuss the trial with their family members before making a decision. In cases

where participants wished to defer to family elders, the research team held family meetings to explain the study and answer questions from both the participant and their relatives.

Outcome:

With these measures in place, the trial successfully enrolled participants while maintaining ethical standards for informed consent. The use of interpreters and audio consent forms significantly improved participant understanding, and the family-focused approach ensured that participants felt supported and confident in their decisions.

CHAPTER 5: PARTICIPANT RECRUITMENT AND RETENTION

Recruiting and retaining participants in clinical trials is one of the most critical and challenging aspects of the trial journey. Effective recruitment ensures that the study reaches its required sample size within the desired timeline, while retention strategies minimize dropouts, preserving the integrity of the trial data.

Practical Strategies for Recruitment

Successful participant recruitment requires a well-structured approach that considers various factors such as the study design, target population, timelines, and site-specific challenges. Below are key strategies that can help improve recruitment outcomes:

1. Defining And Understanding The Target Population

- **Inclusion/Exclusion Criteria**: A clearly defined target population with specific inclusion and exclusion criteria is essential for ensuring that participants are suitable for the trial. These criteria should balance the need for participant safety, relevance to the trial objectives, and ease of recruitment.
- **Feasibility Assessment**: Conduct a feasibility study to evaluate whether the proposed sites have access to the target population and if the recruitment goals are realistic. This process includes analyzing patient databases, assessing site capabilities, and gauging investigator enthusiasm.

2. Developing A Recruitment Plan

- **Timeline Management**: Recruitment timelines must be carefully planned, with clear milestones. Delays in recruitment can impact study timelines and budget, so it is essential to have contingency plans in place.
- **Engagement with Local Communities**: Working closely with local healthcare providers, community leaders, and patient advocacy groups can boost trust and facilitate recruitment, especially in diverse or hard-to-reach populations. This is especially important in studies involving underserved populations or those with limited access to healthcare.
- **Utilizing Digital Tools**: Digital platforms such as social media, clinical trial registries, and online patient forums have become increasingly popular for reaching potential participants. Targeted advertising on these platforms can help identify and recruit participants who meet the study criteria.
- **Collaborating with Primary Care Providers**: Establishing relationships with local healthcare providers who can identify eligible patients and refer them to the study is a highly effective recruitment strategy. This collaborative approach can foster trust and help build a pipeline of potential participants.

3. Recruiting A Diverse Participant Pool

- **Diversity in Clinical Trials**: Ensuring that trials include participants from diverse demographic groups (e.g., age, gender, ethnicity) is crucial for generating results that are applicable to the general population. Tailoring recruitment strategies to address barriers to participation in underrepresented groups can help

improve diversity.
- **Cultural Competence**: Recruiting participants from different cultural backgrounds requires sensitivity to cultural beliefs and practices. This may involve modifying recruitment materials, using bilingual staff, or involving community leaders to encourage participation.
- **Reducing Barriers to Participation**: Common barriers such as travel distance, time commitments, and financial burdens can discourage participants from enrolling. Providing transportation, flexible scheduling, and compensation for time and expenses can significantly enhance recruitment efforts.

4. Incentives And Benefits

- **Monetary Compensation**: Offering compensation for time and travel is a widely accepted practice, but it is important to ensure that the incentive is appropriate and does not influence participants' decision to join the trial for financial reasons.
- **Perceived Benefits**: Clear communication about potential benefits, such as access to cutting-edge treatments or improved healthcare monitoring, can be a strong motivator for participation. However, it is equally important to manage expectations and provide a balanced view of risks and benefits.

Addressing Dropouts And Retention Challenges

Participant retention is just as important as recruitment. High dropout rates can undermine the validity of the trial and lead to incomplete data sets, requiring additional resources to recruit new participants or extend the study. Below are strategies to address common retention challenges:

1. Building Trust And Rapport

- **Clear Communication**: Maintaining open, transparent communication with participants from the start helps build trust and reduces the risk of dropouts. Participants should be fully informed about study progress, potential risks, and their ongoing role in the study.
- **Participant-Centric Approach**: Taking the time to understand each participant's individual needs, preferences, and concerns can make them feel valued. A participant-centric approach, where study coordinators engage with participants regularly, improves retention.

2. Managing Participant Expectations

- **Setting Realistic Expectations**: It is important to set realistic expectations about the study's requirements (e.g., number of visits, tests, and follow-up periods). Unrealistic expectations may lead to participant frustration and increase dropout rates.
- **Explaining the Importance of Commitment**: Educating participants about the importance of completing the trial and how their participation contributes to scientific and medical advances can motivate them to stay engaged.

3. Reducing Participant Burden

- **Flexibility in Scheduling**: Participants often withdraw from trials due to the burden of frequent or inconvenient study visits. Offering flexible visit times, home visits, or remote monitoring options can help alleviate these challenges.

- **Minimizing Invasive Procedures**: Participants may find certain procedures (e.g., blood draws, biopsies) unpleasant, leading to dropouts. Investigators should minimize the number of invasive procedures or clearly explain why they are necessary.

4. Offering Ongoing Support

- **Dedicated Support Team**: Assigning participants a point of contact, such as a clinical trial coordinator, who can provide support throughout the trial can significantly reduce dropouts. This person should be accessible to answer questions, provide updates, and help with logistical issues.
- **Patient Engagement Tools**: Utilizing tools such as patient portals, mobile apps, or SMS reminders can help keep participants informed and engaged. These tools can be used to remind participants of upcoming visits, provide study updates, and encourage adherence to trial protocols.

Case Study: Managing Poor Patient Recruitment In A Multi-Site Trial

Background:
A multi-site, phase III clinical trial was initiated to evaluate a novel treatment for a rare autoimmune disorder. The trial involved 15 sites across three countries. After six months, recruitment was lagging significantly behind schedule, with only 30% of the targeted enrollment achieved.

Some sites had not recruited any participants, while others struggled to reach even a handful of enrollments.

Challenges:
1. **Site-Specific Issues**: Some sites reported difficulty accessing the target population, while others faced competition from similar trials recruiting for the same condition. Certain sites also had limited experience in recruiting for rare diseases, and recruitment staff were unfamiliar with the specific patient needs.
2. **Inadequate Engagement with Local Communities**: In one of the countries, there was a lack of community engagement, and potential participants were hesitant to enroll in a trial they did not fully understand.
3. **Limited Diversity in Recruitment**: Despite the trial being conducted in multiple countries, most participants were from one demographic group, raising concerns about the generalizability of the trial results.

Actions Taken:
1. **Site-Specific Recruitment Plans**: The trial sponsor collaborated with each site to develop tailored recruitment strategies based on local patient populations and healthcare practices. Sites with limited experience in rare disease recruitment were provided with additional training and resources, while high-performing sites were allocated more resources to boost their efforts.
2. **Increased Community Engagement**: The sponsor engaged with local healthcare providers and patient advocacy groups to raise awareness about the trial. These efforts included town hall meetings, educational sessions, and partnerships with community organizations to address concerns and provide potential participants with reliable information.
3. **Expanding Recruitment Efforts**: Digital marketing

campaigns targeting diverse populations were launched to reach potential participants who may not have been identified through traditional healthcare channels. Advertisements were placed on social media, and patient-friendly websites were created to provide more information about the trial.

Outcome:

Within three months, recruitment numbers significantly improved, reaching 75% of the target. The digital campaign attracted more diverse participants, helping to address concerns about the lack of diversity in the trial population.

Furthermore, the site-specific recruitment plans improved the overall efficiency of the trial, and some underperforming sites began to enroll participants at a much higher rate.

CHAPTER 6: CONDUCTING THE TRIAL: DAY-TO-DAY OPERATIONS

Day-to-day operations during a clinical trial require careful management to ensure that data collection, documentation, and overall study conduct are compliant with Good Clinical Practice (GCP) guidelines. From maintaining accurate and complete source documentation to properly addressing and reporting protocol deviations and violations, each operational detail is critical to the trial's success.

GCP-Compliant Data Collection and Documentation

Accurate and complete data collection is the cornerstone of any clinical trial. GCP mandates that all data be recorded, handled, and stored in a way that allows accurate reporting, interpretation, and verification. This ensures the reliability and validity of the trial's results.

1. Source Documentation

Source documents are the original records where trial data is first captured. They are vital for verifying that the clinical trial data reported in the Case Report Forms (CRFs) are accurate and consistent. Source documents include patient medical records, laboratory reports, ECG printouts, and patient-reported outcomes, among others.

- **Key Principles of Source Documentation**:
    - **Attribution**: Every entry in the source document should be attributable to the person who made it, with signatures, initials, or electronic identification.

- **Accuracy and Completeness**: All clinical trial information must be recorded fully, accurately, and promptly. Gaps or inconsistencies in documentation can lead to data queries and may affect the validity of the trial results.
- **Legibility**: Documentation must be clear and readable. Illegible handwriting or ambiguous notes can complicate data review during audits and inspections.
- **Corrections**: If a correction is necessary, it should be made by crossing out the incorrect entry with a single line, entering the correct information, and adding the date, reason for the correction, and the person making the correction.

2. Case Report Forms (Crfs)

The CRF is a tool used to collect all clinical data required by the study protocol. Data entered in the CRF must directly reflect the information from the source documents.

- **CRF Design**: A well-designed CRF is essential for ensuring that data is captured efficiently and accurately. CRFs should include only necessary data fields, ensuring that all required information is collected without unnecessary complexity.
- **Electronic CRFs (eCRFs)**: Increasingly, trials utilize electronic systems for data capture. These systems offer advantages in terms of accuracy, real-time data entry, and audit trails, but they also require rigorous validation to ensure data security and integrity.
- **Data Entry Timeliness**: It is crucial that CRFs are

completed in a timely manner. Delays in data entry can lead to data discrepancies, and missing or late data may affect the trial's outcomes or integrity during regulatory reviews.

Managing Protocol Deviations and Violations

Despite the best efforts to follow the trial protocol, deviations are inevitable in many clinical trials. The challenge lies in identifying, managing, and reporting these deviations in a way that ensures compliance with GCP and minimizes the impact on the trial's integrity.

1. Understanding Protocol Deviations Vs. Violations

- **Protocol Deviation**: A protocol deviation is a departure from the approved protocol that does not significantly affect the participant's rights, safety, or the trial's scientific validity. Examples include a missed visit due to patient scheduling conflicts or minor timing issues with study procedures.
- **Protocol Violation**: A protocol violation, on the other hand, is a more serious breach of the protocol that may affect the participant's rights, safety, or the reliability of the trial data. Examples include enrolling an ineligible participant or failing to follow critical safety monitoring procedures.

2. Preventing Protocol Deviations

- **Training the Study Team**: Ensuring that the entire study team understands the protocol thoroughly is one of the best ways to minimize deviations. Regular training sessions, protocol summaries, and access to FAQs can help the team stay aligned with protocol

requirements.
- **Site Monitoring**: Ongoing site monitoring, both remote and on-site, plays a critical role in identifying and addressing potential issues before they escalate. Monitors review source documents, CRFs, and other trial records to ensure compliance and catch deviations early.

3. Reporting And Managing Deviations

- **Deviation Log**: Every deviation, regardless of its impact, should be recorded in a deviation log. This log should include a description of the deviation, its cause, and the corrective and preventive actions taken. Regular review of the deviation log helps identify patterns and areas for improvement.
- **Immediate Reporting for Serious Violations**: Serious protocol violations that affect participant safety or data integrity must be reported immediately to the sponsor, the institutional review board (IRB), and regulatory authorities. These violations may require immediate corrective actions and could lead to amendments to the protocol.

4. Corrective And Preventive Actions (Capa)

When deviations occur, it's essential to not only correct the immediate issue but also implement preventive measures to avoid recurrence. CAPA plans may include retraining the study team, revising study processes, or implementing additional monitoring.

Case Study: Handling And Reporting Protocol Deviations During An Audit

Background:
A large, multi-site clinical trial was in its final stages when the sponsor was notified of an upcoming regulatory audit. In preparation for the audit, the sponsor conducted an internal audit across the trial sites.

During this internal review, several protocol deviations were identified, ranging from minor deviations to one serious violation that had not been reported to the IRB.

The Protocol Deviations Identified:

1. **Missed Visits**: At two sites, a few participants missed scheduled study visits due to travel difficulties, but the missed visits were not reported as deviations. These deviations were relatively minor and did not impact the trial's safety or validity.

2. **Unreported Dose Adjustment**: In one participant, the study drug dosage had been reduced for two weeks without prior approval or documentation in the protocol amendment. This was a serious protocol violation because the dose adjustment had the potential to affect both participant safety and data reliability.

3. **Delayed Data Entry**: At another site, source documentation was accurate, but CRF entries were delayed for up to six weeks. This delay could compromise data integrity and had not been previously flagged.

Actions Taken:

- **Deviation Reporting**: The sponsor immediately updated the deviation log to reflect all unreported deviations and violations. The serious violation (unapproved dose adjustment) was reported to the IRB and the regulatory authority within 24 hours, and corrective measures were implemented.

- **CAPA Implementation**: The sites involved were

retrained on deviation reporting and protocol adherence. Additionally, the trial sites were required to implement a new system for more timely CRF data entry, with regular monitoring checks to ensure compliance.

- **Audit Outcome**: During the official regulatory audit, the auditors were satisfied with the sponsor's proactive identification and management of the deviations. The CAPA plan was found to be comprehensive, and no further action was required.

Lessons Learned:

- **Proactive Auditing**: Regular internal audits help identify deviations early and prevent serious issues from compromising the trial.
- **Timely Reporting**: Even minor deviations should be reported promptly to ensure transparency and compliance.
- **CAPA Plans**: Effective corrective and preventive actions ensure that deviations are not repeated and the integrity of the trial is preserved.

CHAPTER 7: ADVERSE EVENTS AND SAFETY REPORTING

The safety of trial participants is paramount in clinical research. One of the key components of ensuring participant safety is the identification, documentation, and reporting of adverse events (AEs) and serious adverse events (SAEs). This chapter focuses on the practical applications of safety reporting, risk management, and a case study highlighting challenges related to late SAE reporting.

Identifying and Reporting Adverse Events (AEs) and Serious Adverse Events (SAEs)

Adverse events are any undesirable experiences associated with the use of a drug or intervention in a patient, while serious adverse events are those that result in significant medical outcomes, including death, hospitalization, or persistent disability. Understanding the nuances of identifying and reporting these events is essential for compliance with Good Clinical Practice (GCP) and regulatory requirements.

1. Identifying Adverse Events

- **Definition of Adverse Events**: An AE is any unfavorable or unintended sign, symptom, or disease associated with the use of a medicinal product, whether or not it is related to the treatment.
- **Determining Seriousness**: An SAE is defined by its seriousness, not its severity. An event is considered

serious if it:
- Results in death.
- Is life-threatening.
- Requires hospitalization or prolongation of existing hospitalization.
- Results in persistent or significant disability/incapacity.
- Is a congenital anomaly or birth defect.
- Any other significant medical event that may jeopardize the patient.

2. Reporting Adverse Events And Serious Adverse Events

- **Timeliness**: AEs must be reported promptly according to the protocols set out in the trial design. SAEs, particularly those that are unexpected, must be reported within 24 hours to the sponsor and relevant regulatory authorities.
- **Documentation**: Each AE or SAE should be documented with sufficient detail, including:
  - Description of the event.
  - Date of onset and resolution.
  - Severity and relatedness to the investigational product.
  - Action taken (e.g., drug withdrawal, intervention).
  - Outcome.
- **Use of Standardized Forms**: Many sponsors provide standardized AE and SAE report forms to ensure consistency and completeness in reporting. Utilizing these forms streamlines the reporting process and reduces the risk of missing critical information.

3. Safety Reporting Requirements

- **Regulatory Guidelines**: Adverse event reporting requirements vary by country and regulatory authority. Understanding these guidelines is crucial to ensure compliance and timely reporting. For example, the FDA mandates that serious and unexpected adverse events must be reported within specific timelines.
- **IRB Notification**: Any serious adverse event that impacts participant safety must also be reported to the Institutional Review Board (IRB) promptly, ensuring that ethical oversight is maintained throughout the trial.

Risk Management And Mitigation In Trials

Managing risks associated with adverse events is a critical part of clinical trial oversight. Effective risk management strategies help ensure participant safety and the integrity of trial data.

1. Risk Assessment

- **Identifying Risks**: The trial protocol should include a thorough risk assessment identifying potential AEs and SAEs related to the intervention. This involves considering the drug's mechanism of action, previous clinical data, and patient population characteristics.
- **Regular Monitoring**: Ongoing monitoring of participant safety data throughout the trial can help identify trends or patterns that may indicate a safety concern. This monitoring includes reviewing reported AEs, evaluating laboratory results, and assessing vital signs.

2. Risk Mitigation Strategies

- **Informed Consent Process**: Clear communication about potential risks during the informed consent process helps ensure participants are aware of possible AEs and are engaged in their safety.
- **Safety Monitoring Committees**: Establishing independent safety monitoring committees can provide an additional layer of oversight, ensuring that risks are appropriately assessed and managed.
- **Adaptations to Protocol**: If a concerning trend in AEs is identified, the trial protocol may need to be modified to enhance participant safety, such as implementing additional exclusion criteria or changing dosing regimens.

Case Study: A Challenging Scenario With Late Sae Reporting

Background:
A phase III clinical trial evaluating a new oncology drug was nearing its conclusion when an unexpected serious adverse event (SAE) occurred. One participant experienced a severe allergic reaction, leading to hospitalization and significant morbidity.

Details of the SAE:

- The reaction developed three days after the participant received the investigational drug. The participant was hospitalized for observation and treatment, but the site did not report the SAE to the sponsor for ten days.

Challenges Encountered:

1. **Delayed Reporting**: The research coordinator at the site was unsure whether the event qualified as an SAE and delayed reporting while gathering additional

information from the medical team. This delay led to missed deadlines for regulatory reporting.

2. **Impact on Patient Safety**: The late reporting of the SAE meant that data regarding potential allergic reactions was not available for review during ongoing safety monitoring, potentially jeopardizing participant safety in other sites where similar reactions could occur.

3. **Regulatory Compliance Issues**: The late reporting raised compliance concerns during a subsequent regulatory inspection, as the sponsor had not been informed in a timely manner.

Actions Taken:

- **Immediate Investigation**: Upon learning of the SAE, the sponsor conducted a thorough investigation, including interviews with the site staff and a review of the participant's medical records.
- **Staff Training**: The sponsor organized a retraining session for all site staff on the importance of timely SAE reporting and the specific criteria that classify an event as serious.
- **Updated Reporting Protocol**: A new protocol for SAE reporting was developed, including clear timelines and responsibilities for reporting events. This protocol mandated immediate notification to the medical monitor and expedited the review process for potential SAEs.

Outcome: The late reporting led to significant corrective actions, including improved training and protocols at the site. In subsequent audits, compliance with reporting requirements showed marked improvement, reducing the risk of similar occurrences in future trials.

Lessons Learned:

- **Importance of Clarity**: Clear definitions and training on what constitutes an SAE can prevent delays in reporting.
- **Proactive Monitoring**: Ongoing monitoring and communication channels between sites and sponsors can help identify potential safety issues early and facilitate timely reporting.
- **Stakeholder Engagement**: Engaging all stakeholders in the safety reporting process, including investigators, monitors, and regulatory bodies, fosters a culture of safety and compliance.

CHAPTER 8: MONITORING CLINICAL TRIALS

Monitoring is a critical component of clinical trials, ensuring compliance with Good Clinical Practice (GCP) and regulatory requirements, while safeguarding participant safety and data integrity. This chapter outlines practical approaches to both on-site and remote monitoring, common pitfalls in the monitoring process, and a case study highlighting challenges related to incomplete documentation during a monitoring visit.

Practical Approach to On-Site and Remote Monitoring

Monitoring can be conducted through various methods, including traditional on-site visits and modern remote monitoring techniques. A risk-based approach to monitoring optimizes resources while maintaining participant safety and data quality.

1. On-Site Monitoring

- **Purpose**: On-site monitoring involves physical visits to trial sites to review documentation, observe procedures, and interact with the investigative team. The goals are to ensure compliance, verify data integrity, and assess participant safety.
- **Key Activities**:
    - **Source Data Verification (SDV)**: Confirming the accuracy of data collected by comparing it against original source documents (e.g., patient charts).
    - **Review of Regulatory Documentation**:

Ensuring that essential documents (e.g., IRB approvals, informed consent forms) are current and accessible.
- **Assessing Protocol Compliance**: Observing trial procedures to ensure adherence to the protocol, including recruitment strategies, informed consent processes, and data collection methods.

2. Remote Monitoring

- **Emerging Trend**: Remote monitoring has gained popularity due to advancements in technology and the need for flexibility in clinical trials. It allows for real-time data access and communication without the need for physical site visits.
- **Key Components**:
    - **Use of Electronic Data Capture (EDC)**: EDC systems facilitate real-time data entry and monitoring, enabling immediate access to participant data and reducing delays associated with manual data entry.
    - **Video Conferencing**: Remote meetings between monitors and site staff can help address questions, provide training, and facilitate discussions about participant safety and trial progress.
    - **Centralized Review**: Centralized data monitoring teams can analyze data trends, identify issues, and communicate with sites about potential concerns.

3. Risk-Based Monitoring

- **Definition**: Risk-based monitoring focuses on identifying and prioritizing risks associated with clinical trials. This approach allows monitors to allocate resources effectively and concentrate efforts on areas of highest risk.
- **Implementation**:
  - **Risk Assessment**: Prior to trial initiation, conduct a thorough risk assessment to identify potential challenges, including site capacity, investigator experience, and participant population characteristics.
  - **Ongoing Evaluation**: Continuously evaluate risks throughout the trial, using data analytics and real-time monitoring to identify issues as they arise.
  - **Adaptive Monitoring Plans**: Adjust monitoring strategies based on identified risks, potentially increasing the frequency of visits or implementing targeted remote monitoring for higher-risk sites.

Common Pitfalls In Monitoring And How To Avoid Them

Effective monitoring is essential, but several common pitfalls can hinder the process. Being aware of these challenges can help stakeholders avoid mistakes and enhance the monitoring experience.

1. Incomplete Documentation

- **Issue**: Incomplete or missing documentation is one of the most common issues encountered during monitoring visits. This can include missing informed consent forms, unfilled case report forms (CRFs), or lack of source documentation.

- **Solution**: Establish a robust tracking system to ensure that all required documents are collected and reviewed before monitoring visits. Site staff should be trained on the importance of complete documentation and regular audits should be conducted to identify gaps.

2. Poor Communication

- **Issue**: Ineffective communication between monitors and site staff can lead to misunderstandings regarding protocols, timelines, and responsibilities.
- **Solution**: Foster open lines of communication through regular check-ins, training sessions, and feedback loops. Clearly define expectations and responsibilities for all parties involved.

3. Neglecting Training Needs

- **Issue**: Monitors may overlook the need for ongoing training for site staff, particularly if there are changes to protocols or regulatory requirements.
- **Solution**: Implement regular training sessions, both in-person and remote, to ensure site staff are updated on current practices, regulatory changes, and monitoring expectations.

4. Failing To Document Monitoring Activities

- **Issue**: Monitors may neglect to document their findings and actions taken during monitoring visits, leading to potential compliance issues and lack of accountability.

- **Solution**: Develop standardized templates for monitoring visit reports, ensuring that all findings are documented thoroughly and communicated to relevant stakeholders promptly.

Case Study: Dealing With Incomplete Documentation During A Monitoring Visit

Background:
A clinical trial evaluating a new diabetes medication was underway across multiple sites. During a scheduled on-site monitoring visit, the monitor discovered significant issues with incomplete documentation at one of the trial sites.

Findings:

- Several participants' CRFs were missing essential data points, including laboratory results and concomitant medication information.
- Informed consent forms for two participants were missing signatures, raising concerns about compliance with GCP guidelines.
- Source documents for several AEs had not been recorded properly, creating discrepancies in the safety reporting.

Challenges Encountered:

1. **Impact on Data Integrity**: Incomplete documentation could compromise the integrity of the trial data, making it difficult to assess the safety and efficacy of the investigational product.
2. **Regulatory Compliance Risks**: Missing documents posed a risk of non-compliance with GCP guidelines and regulatory requirements, potentially jeopardizing the trial's credibility.

Actions Taken:

- **Immediate Follow-Up**: The monitor immediately discussed the findings with the site staff, highlighting the importance of complete documentation for maintaining compliance and participant safety.
- **Corrective Action Plan**: A corrective action plan was developed in collaboration with the site staff. This plan included:
    - A timeline for completing missing documentation.
    - Implementing a checklist for site staff to ensure all required documents are collected and reviewed before monitoring visits.
    - Scheduling follow-up training sessions to reinforce the importance of accurate and complete documentation.

Outcome: The site was able to rectify the documentation issues within the specified timeline, and subsequent monitoring visits showed significant improvement in compliance. The corrective action plan not only addressed the immediate concerns but also fostered a culture of accountability and attention to detail among site staff.

Lessons Learned:
- **Proactive Monitoring**: Regularly assessing documentation practices at the site level can help identify issues early and prevent complications during monitoring visits.
- **Collaborative Approach**: Engaging site staff in identifying and resolving documentation challenges fosters a collaborative atmosphere, improving overall compliance.
- **Ongoing Training**: Continuous training and resources for site staff are essential to ensure understanding and adherence to documentation requirements.

CHAPTER 9: QUALITY MANAGEMENT AND AUDITS

Quality management is integral to the success of clinical trials, ensuring that they are conducted in compliance with Good Clinical Practice (GCP) and regulatory requirements while maintaining the highest standards of data integrity and participant safety.

Quality Assurance (QA) vs. Quality Control (QC)

Understanding the distinction between QA and QC is crucial for maintaining quality throughout a clinical trial.

1. Quality Assurance (Qa)

- **Definition**: QA is a proactive process aimed at preventing defects by ensuring that the processes involved in clinical trial operations are well-defined, implemented, and followed. It focuses on establishing systems and procedures to improve the overall quality of the trial.
- **Key Activities**:
    - **Standard Operating Procedures (SOPs)**: Developing and implementing SOPs that outline the processes and protocols for trial operations.
    - **Training**: Ensuring that all personnel involved in the trial are adequately trained on protocols, procedures, and compliance requirements.
    - **Internal Audits**: Conducting regular internal

audits to assess compliance with SOPs, GCP, and regulatory requirements, identifying areas for improvement.

2. Quality Control (Qc)

- **Definition**: QC is a reactive process that involves the identification and correction of defects in trial operations. It focuses on monitoring the outputs of processes to ensure they meet the required standards.
- **Key Activities**:
    - **Data Verification**: Regularly reviewing and verifying collected data to ensure accuracy and completeness.
    - **Monitoring Visits**: Conducting on-site monitoring visits to observe trial procedures, verify data against source documents, and ensure compliance with GCP.
    - **Corrective Actions**: Implementing corrective actions when deviations from protocols or quality standards are identified.

Practical Steps For Maintaining Quality Throughout The Trial

Implementing a robust quality management system is essential for maintaining quality throughout the clinical trial journey. Here are practical steps that can be taken:

1. Establish Clear SOPs

- Develop and disseminate clear SOPs for all aspects of the trial, including recruitment, data collection, reporting of adverse events, and monitoring.
- Ensure that all stakeholders are trained on these SOPs and understand their roles and responsibilities.

2. Implement Risk-Based Quality Management
- Conduct a risk assessment during the trial planning phase to identify potential quality risks.
- Prioritize monitoring and quality control activities based on the identified risks, focusing resources on high-risk areas.

3. Engage in Continuous Training
- Provide ongoing training for site staff and monitors to keep them updated on GCP guidelines, regulatory changes, and trial-specific protocols.
- Utilize various training formats, including workshops, webinars, and hands-on training sessions.

4. Conduct Regular Internal Audits
- Schedule regular internal audits to assess compliance with SOPs, GCP, and regulatory requirements.
- Use audit findings to implement corrective actions and improve processes continuously.

5. Foster a Culture of Quality
- Promote a culture that values quality among all trial stakeholders, emphasizing the importance of adherence to protocols and procedures.
- Encourage open communication regarding quality concerns, enabling stakeholders to raise issues without fear of repercussions.

Preparing For Audits And Inspections

Preparation for audits and inspections is crucial for ensuring compliance with regulatory requirements and maintaining the integrity of the trial. Here are key steps to prepare effectively:

1. Understand the Regulatory Requirements
- Familiarize yourself with the specific regulatory requirements relevant to the trial, including GCP

guidelines and local regulations.
- Ensure that all team members understand their roles and responsibilities during audits and inspections.

2. Maintain Comprehensive Documentation
- Ensure that all trial-related documentation is complete, organized, and readily accessible. This includes source documents, CRFs, informed consent forms, and regulatory submissions.
- Implement a document management system to track and manage trial documents effectively.

3. Conduct Mock Audits
- Perform mock audits to simulate the audit process and identify areas of improvement.
- Use findings from mock audits to address potential issues and enhance compliance.

4. Designate a Point of Contact
- Appoint a designated point of contact to interact with auditors during the inspection process. This individual should be knowledgeable about the trial and its documentation.
- Ensure that this person is available during the audit and can address auditor inquiries effectively.

Case Study: Navigating A Gcp Audit From The Fda

Background:
A mid-sized pharmaceutical company was conducting a Phase II clinical trial for a new cardiovascular medication. The FDA announced an upcoming audit to review the trial's compliance with GCP.

Preparation:

- **Pre-Audit Meeting**: The clinical trial team held a pre-audit meeting to review the audit scope, roles, and responsibilities.
- **Document Review**: Team members conducted a thorough review of all documentation, ensuring that all source documents, CRFs, and regulatory submissions were complete and up to date.
- **Mock Audit**: The team organized a mock audit to identify potential issues and rehearse responses to common audit questions.

The Audit Process:

- **Opening Meeting**: The FDA auditors conducted an opening meeting with the trial team to outline the audit process and expectations.
- **On-Site Review**: Auditors reviewed participant files, source documents, and CRFs, verifying data accuracy and compliance with protocols.
- **Interviews with Site Staff**: Auditors conducted interviews with site staff to assess their understanding of protocols, GCP guidelines, and their roles in the trial.

Findings:

- **Positive Outcomes**: The audit identified areas of strong compliance, including well-maintained documentation and effective participant management processes.
- **Minor Deviations**: Some minor deviations were noted, such as incomplete documentation for a few adverse events. The team was able to provide corrective action plans for these issues.

Post-Audit Actions:

- **Corrective Action Plan**: Following the audit, the team developed a corrective action plan to address the identified deviations, implementing additional

training for site staff.
- **Continuous Improvement**: The audit results were used to enhance internal processes and training, fostering a culture of quality and compliance.

Lessons Learned:
- **Preparation is Key**: Thorough preparation, including document reviews and mock audits, significantly contributed to the trial's successful navigation of the audit.
- **Collaboration and Communication**: Open communication among team members ensured that everyone understood their roles and responsibilities during the audit process.
- **Ongoing Quality Management**: Regular audits and internal reviews are essential for maintaining quality and ensuring compliance throughout the trial.

CHAPTER 10: DATA MANAGEMENT AND INTEGRITY

Data management and integrity are paramount in clinical trials, as they directly affect the validity of the trial results and the safety of participants.

Best Practices For Ensuring Data Integrity

Ensuring data integrity involves maintaining the accuracy, completeness, and reliability of data throughout the clinical trial process. Here are best practices for achieving this goal, particularly focusing on the practical application of electronic data capture (EDC) systems and databases.

1. **Utilize Electronic Data Capture (EDC) Systems**
   - **Implementation of EDC Systems**: Utilize EDC systems for real-time data entry, reducing transcription errors and improving data quality. These systems allow for immediate data validation checks and automated audit trails.
   - **User Training**: Provide comprehensive training for all users on how to operate the EDC system effectively, ensuring they understand data entry processes, validation rules, and how to handle system alerts.
   - **System Validation**: Ensure that the EDC system is validated according to regulatory requirements, demonstrating that it performs as intended and produces reliable data.

2. **Maintain Comprehensive Data Entry Protocols**
   - **Standardized Data Entry**: Develop standardized data entry protocols to ensure consistency in how data

is recorded. This includes defining data formats, terminology, and codes to be used.

- **Source Data Verification (SDV)**: Regularly conduct SDV to ensure that the data entered into the EDC system accurately reflects the source documents, such as case report forms (CRFs) and medical records.

3. **Implement Data Monitoring and Auditing Procedures**

- **Regular Data Monitoring**: Conduct regular data monitoring to identify and address discrepancies or trends that may indicate data integrity issues. Utilize statistical methods to assess data completeness and consistency.
- **Audits**: Schedule routine audits of data management processes to ensure compliance with SOPs and regulatory requirements. Focus on high-risk areas where data integrity may be compromised.

4. **Employ Robust Security Measures**

- **Access Controls**: Implement strict access controls to limit who can view or edit data in the EDC system. Use role-based access to ensure that only authorized personnel can make changes.
- **Data Encryption**: Use encryption to protect data during transmission and storage, ensuring that sensitive participant information remains confidential.

Handling Missing Data And Queries

Missing data is a common challenge in clinical trials, and effectively managing it is essential to maintain the integrity of the study results. Here are strategies for handling missing data and addressing queries:

1. **Proactive Missing Data Management**

- **Identify Potential Causes**: At the trial design stage,

identify potential sources of missing data, such as participant dropout or incomplete responses. Develop strategies to minimize these occurrences.

- **Monitoring for Missing Data**: Continuously monitor data for missing entries, using real-time data analysis tools within the EDC system to flag missing values and generate alerts for follow-up.

2. Addressing Missing Data

- **Data Imputation**: Use appropriate statistical methods to handle missing data, such as data imputation techniques. This allows for the inclusion of incomplete data while minimizing bias in analysis.
- **Documentation**: Document the reasons for missing data, how it was addressed, and the impact on the study's findings in the final report. Transparency in how missing data was handled is critical for maintaining credibility.

3. Query Management

- **Timely Query Resolution**: Establish a systematic process for generating and resolving data queries. Queries should be resolved promptly to ensure the accuracy of the data.
- **Clear Communication**: Ensure clear communication between data managers, site staff, and investigators regarding data queries. Provide guidance on how to address specific data issues and what information is required.

Case Study: Data Discrepancies In A Blinded Trial And How They Were Resolved

Background:
A multinational pharmaceutical company conducted a double-blind Phase III clinical trial to evaluate the efficacy of a new

medication for managing hypertension. During the trial, data discrepancies were identified in the EDC system, raising concerns about the integrity of the data.

Initial Discovery:

- **Routine Monitoring**: During routine monitoring, the data management team noted inconsistencies between the EDC entries and the source documents, particularly concerning blood pressure readings recorded by site investigators.
- **Discrepancy Report**: The team generated a discrepancy report, highlighting the inconsistencies and the affected participants. The discrepancies included variations in readings that were outside the expected ranges based on prior visits.

Investigation Process:

- **Site Engagement**: The data management team reached out to the involved trial sites to investigate the discrepancies. Site staff were asked to review their records and provide explanations for the inconsistencies.
- **Data Reconciliation**: A reconciliation process was initiated, involving side-by-side comparisons of the EDC data with the source documents. This process helped identify errors in data entry and issues related to the timing of blood pressure assessments.

Resolution:

- **Corrective Actions**: After identifying the root causes of the discrepancies, corrective actions were implemented. Site staff received additional training on accurate data entry and the importance of timely data reporting.
- **Adjustment of Data**: Data entries in the EDC system were adjusted based on the verified source data. In cases where it was determined that data were missing

or inaccurately recorded, appropriate imputation techniques were employed to minimize bias.

Lessons Learned:

- **Importance of Real-Time Monitoring**: The incident highlighted the need for real-time monitoring of data integrity throughout the trial. Early identification of discrepancies allowed for timely interventions.
- **Strengthening Training Programs**: The trial emphasized the importance of ongoing training for site staff to ensure they understand data entry processes and the critical nature of accurate reporting.
- **Collaboration is Key**: Effective collaboration between the data management team and site staff was crucial in resolving discrepancies and ensuring the integrity of the trial data.

CHAPTER 11: INVESTIGATIONAL MEDICINAL PRODUCT (IMP) MANAGEMENT

Effective management of Investigational Medicinal Products (IMPs) is critical for the success of clinical trials.

1. Understanding IMP Management

IMPs are products being tested or used as a reference in a clinical trial, including pharmaceuticals, biologics, or any other substances administered to trial participants. Proper management of these products is essential to ensure participant safety, data integrity, and regulatory compliance.

Key Components Of Imp Management

- **Preparation**: The preparation of IMPs must follow established protocols to ensure consistency, quality, and safety. This includes compounding, labeling, and packaging according to regulatory guidelines.
- **Storage**: IMPs must be stored under specified conditions to maintain their stability and efficacy. This includes temperature control, protection from light, and security measures to prevent unauthorized access.
- **Distribution**: Efficient distribution channels must be established to ensure timely delivery of IMPs to trial sites while maintaining appropriate documentation for tracking and accountability.
- **Accountability and Documentation**: Detailed records

must be maintained at every stage of the IMP lifecycle, from preparation and storage to distribution and return. This includes inventory logs, shipping records, and accountability forms.

2. Regulatory Considerations For Imp Management

To ensure compliance with GCP and regulatory requirements, several key considerations must be addressed in IMP management:

- **Regulatory Compliance**: IMPs must comply with relevant regulations, including those set forth by the Food and Drug Administration (FDA), European Medicines Agency (EMA), or other local regulatory bodies. This includes adhering to Good Manufacturing Practices (GMP) and labeling requirements.
- **Investigator Responsibilities**: Investigators are responsible for the proper handling of IMPs at the trial site. This includes ensuring that study staff are trained in IMP management, monitoring compliance with storage conditions, and maintaining accurate records.
- **Monitoring by Sponsors and CROs**: Sponsors and Contract Research Organizations (CROs) must implement monitoring plans to ensure that IMP management procedures are followed throughout the trial. This includes regular audits and site visits to verify compliance with GCP standards.

3. Challenges in IMP Management

Effective IMP management can encounter several challenges, including:

- **Temperature Excursions**: Deviations from prescribed storage conditions can compromise the integrity of IMPs, necessitating immediate corrective actions and

documentation.
- **Supply Chain Issues**: Disruptions in the supply chain can lead to delays in IMP availability at trial sites, impacting recruitment and participant retention.
- **Handling and Accountability**: Mismanagement of IMPs can lead to accountability issues, such as loss or mislabeling of products, which can compromise trial integrity and participant safety.

4. Best Practices For Imp Management

To overcome challenges and ensure effective IMP management, the following best practices should be implemented:
- **Standard Operating Procedures (SOPs)**: Develop and implement comprehensive SOPs for all aspects of IMP management, including preparation, storage, and distribution.
- **Training**: Provide regular training for all personnel involved in IMP management to ensure they understand their roles, responsibilities, and the importance of compliance with GCP and regulatory requirements.
- **Monitoring and Auditing**: Establish a robust monitoring and auditing framework to regularly assess IMP management practices, identify potential issues, and implement corrective actions promptly.
- **Contingency Planning**: Develop contingency plans to address potential supply chain disruptions or temperature excursions, including protocols for alternate storage and retrieval options.

Case Study: Managing Investigational Medicinal Products In A Multicenter Clinical Trial

Background:
A pharmaceutical company initiated a multicenter clinical trial to evaluate a new antihypertensive medication. The trial involved multiple sites across different regions, requiring meticulous IMP management to ensure compliance with GCP and regulatory standards.

Challenges Faced:
1. **Temperature Excursion**: During the trial, it was reported that an IMP shipment to one of the sites experienced a temperature excursion, raising concerns about the product's integrity.
2. **Delays in Supply Chain**: A delay in the supply of the IMP from the manufacturer caused disruptions in recruitment efforts at several trial sites.
3. **Accountability Issues**: At one site, discrepancies were found in the inventory logs, leading to confusion about the number of IMPs available for participants.

Strategies Implemented:
1. **Immediate Action on Temperature Excursion**: Upon receiving the report of the temperature excursion, the trial manager conducted an immediate investigation. The affected batch was quarantined, and the manufacturer was consulted to assess the product's stability. After confirming that the IMP remained within acceptable limits, it was released for use with appropriate documentation.
2. **Supply Chain Management**: The sponsor established a direct line of communication with the manufacturer and logistics providers to anticipate potential delays. A contingency plan was implemented, including the

identification of alternative suppliers and expedited shipping options to minimize impact on trial timelines.
3. **Strengthening Accountability**: To address accountability issues, the trial team introduced electronic inventory management systems at all sites. This system allowed for real-time tracking of IMPs, reducing the likelihood of discrepancies and improving overall transparency.

Outcome:
- **Successful Trial Continuation**: The proactive measures taken to address temperature excursions and supply chain delays minimized disruptions to the trial timeline, allowing recruitment goals to be met effectively.
- **Improved Data Integrity**: The introduction of electronic inventory management improved accountability and data integrity, ensuring accurate tracking of IMPs throughout the trial.
- **Enhanced Compliance**: Continuous training and monitoring ensured that all site staff were well-versed in GCP requirements, leading to successful compliance during regulatory audits.

Conclusion

Effective IMP management is critical to the success of clinical trials, impacting participant safety, data integrity, and overall trial compliance. By implementing best practices, adhering to regulatory guidelines, and addressing challenges proactively, stakeholders can ensure that IMPs are managed efficiently and responsibly. The case study illustrates the importance of meticulous planning, communication, and adaptability in overcoming obstacles in IMP management, reinforcing the need for continuous improvement in

ESSAM ABDELHAKIM

clinical research practices.

CHAPTER 12: CLOSING A CLINICAL TRIAL

Closing a clinical trial is a critical phase that involves a series of systematic procedures to ensure that all aspects of the trial are completed in compliance with Good Clinical Practice (GCP) guidelines.

Trial Close-Out Procedures

The trial close-out phase is essential for ensuring that the clinical trial is concluded properly and that all necessary documentation is completed. Here are the key components of the trial close-out procedures:

1. Final Monitoring
   - **Site Visits**: Conduct final monitoring visits to each trial site to ensure that all data have been accurately recorded and that all trial-related activities have been completed. This includes reviewing source documents and confirming that any outstanding queries have been resolved.
   - **Ensuring Compliance**: Verify that sites have adhered to protocol requirements and GCP principles throughout the trial. Address any discrepancies or non-compliance issues identified during the monitoring visits.

2. Data Lock
   - **Final Data Review**: Perform a thorough review of the collected data to ensure completeness and accuracy. Identify any last-minute discrepancies that need to be addressed before locking the data.

- **Data Lock Procedures**: Implement the formal process for data lock, which involves finalizing the dataset and restricting further changes. Document the data lock date and the personnel responsible for approving the lock.
- **Backup and Archiving**: Create backups of the locked data and ensure secure storage. Plan for long-term data archiving in accordance with regulatory requirements.

3. Database Closure
- **Database Cleanup**: Conduct a final cleanup of the database to remove any erroneous or duplicate entries. Ensure that all data fields are populated according to the protocol.
- **Final Checks**: Carry out final checks to confirm that the database aligns with the source documents and that all data entries are complete and accurate.
- **Audit Trail Review**: Review the audit trail of the database to ensure that all changes made during the trial are documented and that proper version control is maintained.

Final Reports And Regulatory Submissions

After the trial has been closed and the data locked, the next steps involve preparing final reports and submitting necessary documentation to regulatory authorities.

1. Final Clinical Study Report (CSR)
- **Report Preparation**: Draft the final Clinical Study Report, which summarizes the trial's objectives, methodology, results, and conclusions. Ensure that the CSR is compliant with regulatory requirements and guidelines.
- **Incorporating Feedback**: Include feedback from stakeholders such as investigators, sponsors, and

regulatory authorities. This collaborative approach ensures that all perspectives are considered in the final report.

- **Statistical Analysis**: Collaborate with biostatisticians to present the statistical analysis of the data clearly. Include relevant tables, figures, and appendices to support the findings.

2. Regulatory Submissions

- **Submission to Regulatory Authorities**: Prepare the necessary documentation for submission to regulatory authorities (e.g., FDA, EMA). This may include the final CSR, investigator brochures, and any additional data required by the regulators.
- **Follow-Up and Responses**: Be prepared to respond to any questions or requests for additional information from regulatory authorities following the submission. Maintain open communication with the relevant agencies to facilitate the review process.

Case Study: Efficiently Closing A Trial With Minimal Errors

Background:

A multinational pharmaceutical company conducted a Phase II clinical trial to evaluate the safety and efficacy of a new treatment for type 2 diabetes. The trial included multiple sites across different countries and involved over 300 participants.

Closing Procedures:

1. **Final Monitoring Visits**: The project manager scheduled final monitoring visits to each site. During these visits, monitors conducted thorough reviews of source documents and EDC entries, ensuring that all data were complete and accurate.
2. **Data Lock Process**: Once all discrepancies were

resolved, the data management team conducted a final data review. They engaged in a collaborative approach with site staff to ensure accuracy. On the agreed date, the data lock was implemented, with all necessary personnel approving the lock.

3. **Database Closure**: The database was then cleaned and validated for accuracy. The team ensured that all relevant data fields were populated and performed final checks to confirm that the database was consistent with the source documents.

Final Reports and Submissions:

- The Clinical Study Report was prepared in accordance with ICH E3 guidelines. The biostatistics team conducted the final analysis and presented the findings in a clear and concise manner. All team members provided feedback on the report, which helped to enhance its quality.
- Regulatory submissions were prepared and submitted to the relevant authorities in a timely manner, including all required documentation and summaries of the trial findings.

Outcome:

- The trial was successfully closed with minimal errors, and all required documentation was submitted within the stipulated timelines. Feedback from regulatory authorities was positive, and the company was able to proceed to the next phase of development for the new treatment.

Lessons Learned:

- **Thorough Preparation**: Comprehensive final monitoring and data review processes were key to minimizing errors during the trial closure. Early identification and resolution of issues contributed to a smooth close-out.

- **Collaboration**: Open communication among all stakeholders facilitated a successful trial closure and timely completion of regulatory submissions.
- **Documentation**: Ensuring meticulous documentation throughout the trial enabled efficient report preparation and regulatory submission, ultimately enhancing the credibility of the findings.

CHAPTER 13: POST-TRIAL CONSIDERATIONS

The post-trial phase is crucial for ensuring that the insights gained from clinical trials are applied effectively to real-world settings.

Post-Marketing Surveillance And Long-Term Safety Monitoring

Post-marketing surveillance refers to the processes in place to monitor the safety and effectiveness of a drug or treatment after it has been approved for general use. Long-term safety monitoring is critical for identifying any adverse effects that may not have been apparent during the clinical trial phase.

1. Importance of Post-Marketing Surveillance
    - **Ongoing Risk Assessment**: Post-marketing surveillance helps identify rare adverse events that may only become apparent when a drug is used in a larger and more diverse population. This ongoing assessment is essential for maintaining patient safety.
    - **Data Collection**: Ongoing data collection through various methods—such as patient registries, electronic health records, and spontaneous reporting systems—provides a wealth of information on the long-term effects of a treatment.

2. Long-Term Safety Monitoring
    - **Follow-Up Studies**: Conducting follow-up studies on trial participants can provide valuable data on the long-term safety and efficacy of a drug. These studies may involve regular health assessments, lab tests, or surveys.

- **Risk Management Plans**: Developing comprehensive risk management plans that outline strategies for minimizing and mitigating risks associated with the drug can enhance safety. This may include risk communication strategies to inform healthcare providers and patients of potential risks.

3. Regulatory Requirements
    - **Compliance with Regulations**: Regulatory authorities often require post-marketing surveillance and long-term safety monitoring as a condition of drug approval. Understanding these requirements and ensuring compliance is essential for maintaining market authorization.

Case Study: Managing Ongoing Safety Monitoring In A Drug Trial After Approval

Background:
A pharmaceutical company developed a novel anticoagulant drug for preventing blood clots. After successful Phase III trials and subsequent approval by regulatory authorities, the company initiated a post-marketing surveillance program to monitor the drug's safety and efficacy in a broader population.

Ongoing Safety Monitoring Procedures:

1. **Establishment of a Patient Registry**: The company set up a patient registry to track long-term outcomes and adverse events in patients taking the new anticoagulant. Healthcare providers were encouraged to report any adverse events experienced by their patients through a dedicated hotline and online portal.

2. **Regular Safety Assessments**: Patients in the registry were scheduled for regular follow-up visits to assess their health status, review any side effects, and conduct laboratory tests to monitor coagulation parameters. These assessments helped identify any trends or emerging safety concerns.
3. **Data Analysis and Reporting**: The safety data collected through the registry were regularly analyzed to identify any patterns of adverse events. Monthly reports were generated, summarizing the findings, which were shared with regulatory authorities and stakeholders.

Outcome:

- The ongoing safety monitoring program identified a rare but significant adverse event—a higher-than-expected incidence of gastrointestinal bleeding in certain patient populations. The company took prompt action to communicate this risk to healthcare providers and patients through a label update and risk communication strategies.
- The proactive approach to safety monitoring allowed the company to maintain trust with regulatory authorities and the public, reinforcing the importance of post-marketing surveillance in drug safety.

Lessons Learned: Key Takeaways for Future Trials

Reflecting on past trials provides an opportunity to improve future practices. Here are some key takeaways that can enhance the quality and safety of future clinical trials:

1. Importance of Continuous Monitoring

- **Implement Robust Monitoring Systems**: Establishing effective monitoring systems from the outset of a clinical trial can help identify issues early and facilitate timely interventions.

2. **Engage Stakeholders Throughout the Process**
    - **Collaborate with Stakeholders**: Involving stakeholders—such as regulatory authorities, healthcare providers, and patients—throughout the trial and post-trial phases fosters transparency and collaboration, leading to better outcomes.
3. **Document and Share Findings**
    - **Create a Culture of Learning**: Thorough documentation of challenges and successes can provide valuable insights for future trials. Sharing these lessons with the broader clinical research community promotes a culture of learning and continuous improvement.

Case Study: Reflecting On Lessons From A Successful Trial To Improve Future Practices

Background:
A biopharmaceutical company conducted a successful trial of a new treatment for a rare genetic disorder, leading to rapid approval and market entry. The team conducted a thorough retrospective analysis of the trial to identify lessons learned for future studies.

Key Lessons Identified:
1. **Strong Patient Engagement**: The trial's success was attributed to effective patient engagement strategies that involved educating participants about the trial process and providing ongoing support. This approach enhanced recruitment and retention rates.
2. **Adaptive Trial Design**: The use of an adaptive trial design allowed for modifications to the trial protocol based on interim results. This flexibility enabled the team to optimize patient outcomes and resource allocation.

3. **Thorough Training of Investigative Teams**: Comprehensive training of investigative teams on protocol adherence and GCP principles contributed to the trial's success. The company recognized the importance of ongoing education and skill development for all team members involved in clinical trials.

Outcome:

- The insights gained from this successful trial informed the planning and execution of future studies. The company implemented a series of training workshops focused on patient engagement and adaptive trial designs, significantly improving the outcomes of subsequent trials.

CHAPTER 14: CASE STUDIES IN GCP APPLICATION

Common Gcp Violations And How To Avoid Them

1. Incomplete Or Inaccurate Documentation

- **Violation**: Missing or incorrectly filled Case Report Forms (CRFs) can lead to data integrity issues and compromise trial results.
- **Avoidance Strategy**: Implement rigorous training programs for investigative staff on the importance of accurate documentation. Utilize electronic data capture systems with built-in validation checks to minimize errors and ensure completeness.

2. Failure To Obtain Informed Consent

- **Violation**: Participants may not fully understand the study, leading to non-compliance with informed consent regulations.
- **Avoidance Strategy**: Develop clear, culturally appropriate consent forms and utilize plain language to explain the study's purpose, risks, and benefits. Conduct training sessions for the investigative team on effective communication techniques, especially for diverse populations.

3. Non-Compliance With Protocol

- **Violation**: Deviations from the approved study protocol can jeopardize data quality and participant safety.
- **Avoidance Strategy**: Regularly review the protocol with the investigative team and implement a robust monitoring plan that includes frequent audits to identify and address deviations proactively.

4. Inadequate Reporting Of Adverse Events

- **Violation**: Delays or failures in reporting adverse events (AEs) and serious adverse events (SAEs) can impact participant safety and regulatory compliance.
- **Avoidance Strategy**: Establish a clear process for identifying, documenting, and reporting AEs and SAEs. Provide training for all team members on the importance of timely reporting and the regulatory requirements for safety monitoring.

5. Insufficient Training Of Investigative Staff

- **Violation**: Lack of adequate training can lead to misunderstandings of GCP guidelines and study protocols.
- **Avoidance Strategy**: Develop comprehensive training programs that cover GCP principles, protocol specifics, and site responsibilities. Use interactive training methods such as simulations and role-playing to enhance understanding and retention.

Case Study: A Multi-Disciplinary Approach To Resolving Gcp Compliance Issues

Background:

A pharmaceutical company was conducting a clinical trial for a new diabetes medication. During a routine monitoring visit, the monitor identified several GCP compliance issues, including incomplete CRFs, inconsistent AE reporting, and lack of proper documentation for informed consent.

Challenges:
- **Inconsistent Data**: The monitoring report highlighted discrepancies in data entries that raised concerns about data integrity.
- **Delays in AE Reporting**: The clinical research coordinator (CRC) had not consistently reported AEs, resulting in potential safety risks for participants.
- **Training Gaps**: The investigative team lacked a thorough understanding of GCP requirements, particularly concerning informed consent and documentation.

Cross-Functional Collaboration Approach:
1. **Establishment of a Compliance Task Force**: The company formed a cross-functional task force that included representatives from clinical operations, regulatory affairs, data management, and the investigative team. The task force aimed to address the identified compliance issues collaboratively.
2. **Comprehensive Training Sessions**: The task force organized training sessions for the investigative team focused on GCP principles, proper documentation practices, and the importance of timely AE reporting. The training emphasized the implications of GCP violations for participant safety and data integrity.
3. **Regular Monitoring and Feedback**: The task force

implemented a robust monitoring system that included bi-weekly audits of documentation and AE reporting. Feedback was provided to the investigative team, allowing for continuous improvement.

4. **Improved Communication Channels**: The task force established regular communication channels among stakeholders, including scheduled meetings and a shared online platform for document review and discussion of compliance concerns.

Outcome:

- **Enhanced Compliance**: The collaborative efforts resulted in a significant reduction in GCP violations, with complete and accurate documentation of CRFs and timely AE reporting becoming the norm.
- **Positive Audit Results**: Subsequent monitoring visits and audits showed marked improvement in compliance, leading to a successful continuation of the trial and building trust with regulatory authorities.
- **Cultural Shift**: The task force's work fostered a culture of accountability and collaboration, emphasizing the importance of GCP compliance throughout the organization.

CHAPTER 15: EMERGING TRENDS IN GCP AND FUTURE DIRECTIONS

The landscape of clinical trials is evolving rapidly, driven by technological advancements and the need for more flexible and patient-centric approaches.

The Role Of Technology In Modern Clinical Trials

As technology continues to advance, its integration into clinical trials offers numerous opportunities to enhance efficiency, improve participant engagement, and ensure compliance with GCP standards.

1. E-Consent
- **Definition**: E-consent is an electronic version of the traditional informed consent process, allowing participants to review, sign, and manage consent documents digitally.
- **Benefits**:
  - **Accessibility**: E-consent improves access to trial information, enabling participants to review consent forms at their convenience and in a setting that feels comfortable.
  - **Engagement**: Interactive e-consent platforms can provide multimedia content (videos, infographics) that enhance understanding of the study.
  - **Real-Time Updates**: Researchers can quickly update consent documents and notify participants of changes, ensuring they have the most current information.

2. Virtual Trials

- **Definition**: Virtual trials (or remote trials) leverage telemedicine and digital tools to conduct clinical research without requiring participants to visit traditional clinical sites.
- **Benefits**:
    - **Flexibility**: Participants can engage in trials from their homes, reducing barriers to participation, especially for those with mobility issues or geographical constraints.
    - **Increased Diversity**: Virtual trials can reach a broader, more diverse population, as participants are not limited by proximity to trial sites.
    - **Real-Time Data Collection**: Wearable devices and mobile apps allow for continuous monitoring and real-time data collection, enhancing the quality of trial data.

3. Artificial Intelligence (Ai) Applications

- **Definition**: AI technologies are increasingly used in various aspects of clinical trials, including participant recruitment, data management, and analysis.
- **Benefits**:
    - **Data Analysis**: AI can analyze large datasets quickly, identifying patterns and insights that can enhance decision-making.
    - **Predictive Modeling**: AI algorithms can predict patient outcomes and optimize trial designs based on historical data, improving efficiency and reducing costs.

- **Automation**: Automating repetitive tasks (e.g., data entry, monitoring) allows researchers to focus on more complex and critical aspects of the trial.

Adapting GCP for Decentralized and Hybrid Trials

As clinical trials become more decentralized, it is essential to adapt GCP guidelines to ensure compliance while embracing these innovative approaches. Here are key considerations for adapting GCP in the context of decentralized and hybrid trials.

1. Regulatory Compliance

- **Continuous Engagement**: Regulatory authorities must engage with stakeholders to establish clear guidelines for decentralized trials, addressing data integrity, participant safety, and informed consent in a virtual environment.
- **Flexible GCP Standards**: GCP standards should evolve to accommodate innovative trial designs while maintaining the core principles of participant protection and data integrity.

2. Data Security and Integrity

- **Cybersecurity Measures**: As trials increasingly rely on digital tools, ensuring robust cybersecurity measures is crucial to protect participant data and maintain integrity.
- **Data Validation**: Implement stringent data validation processes to ensure accuracy and completeness, especially with remote data collection.

3. Training and Support

- **Staff Training**: Provide comprehensive training for investigative teams on new technologies and their implications for GCP compliance. This includes understanding how to utilize e-consent platforms and telehealth tools effectively.

- **Participant Support**: Develop support systems for participants to navigate new technologies, including troubleshooting assistance and access to resources that enhance their understanding of the trial process.

Case Study: Implementing A Decentralized Clinical Trial While Maintaining Gcp Compliance

Background:
A biopharmaceutical company aimed to conduct a decentralized clinical trial for a new migraine treatment. The goal was to enhance participant engagement and diversity while ensuring compliance with GCP standards.

Key Challenges:

- **Ensuring Informed Consent**: The team faced challenges in obtaining informed consent remotely, particularly for participants with varying levels of technological proficiency.
- **Maintaining Data Integrity**: The collection of data through wearables and mobile applications raised concerns regarding data security and integrity.
- **Compliance Monitoring**: The decentralized nature of the trial made it difficult to monitor compliance effectively.

Strategies Implemented:

1. **E-Consent Platform**: The company developed a user-friendly e-consent platform that included video explanations of the study, interactive features, and easy access to ask questions. A helpline was established to assist participants in the consent process.

2. **Telehealth Support**: Investigative teams conducted virtual visits to engage with participants, monitor their progress, and provide support. These visits allowed for real-time assessments of participant well-being and adherence to study protocols.
3. **Data Security Measures**: A robust cybersecurity framework was implemented to protect participant data. This included encryption, secure servers, and regular audits to ensure compliance with data protection regulations.
4. **Continuous Monitoring and Feedback**: The company established a monitoring plan that included regular assessments of compliance and data integrity. Feedback loops were created for both participants and the investigative team to address any issues promptly.

Outcome:

- **Increased Participation**: The decentralized approach led to higher participant engagement and diversity, as individuals from remote locations could participate in the trial.
- **Enhanced Data Quality**: The use of technology for real-time monitoring and data collection resulted in high-quality data while maintaining participant safety and well-being.
- **Successful Compliance**: The proactive measures taken to address GCP compliance challenges led to a successful trial outcome, reinforcing the importance of adapting GCP principles in modern clinical research.

ABOUT THE AUTHOR

Dr Essam Abdelhakim

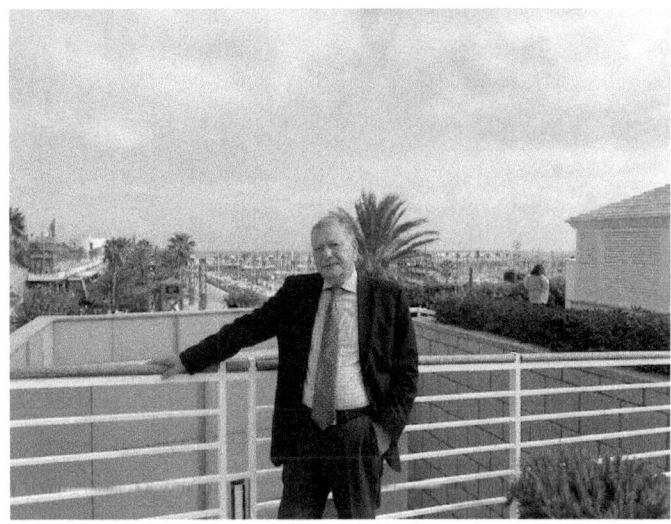

Senior Physician and Expert in Medical Research

www.ingramcontent.com/pod-product-compliance
Lightning Source LLC
Chambersburg PA
CBHW050325230526
45471CB00005B/2348